This publication is intended to provide educational information for the reader on the covered subjects. It is not intended to take the place of personalized medical counseling, diagnosis, and treatment from a trained healthcare professional.

ISBN 978-1-998455-63-8 (Paperback)
ISBN 978-1-998455-64-5 (eBook)

Printed and bound in USA
Published by Loons Press

LOONS PRESS

AF799992

Table Of Contents

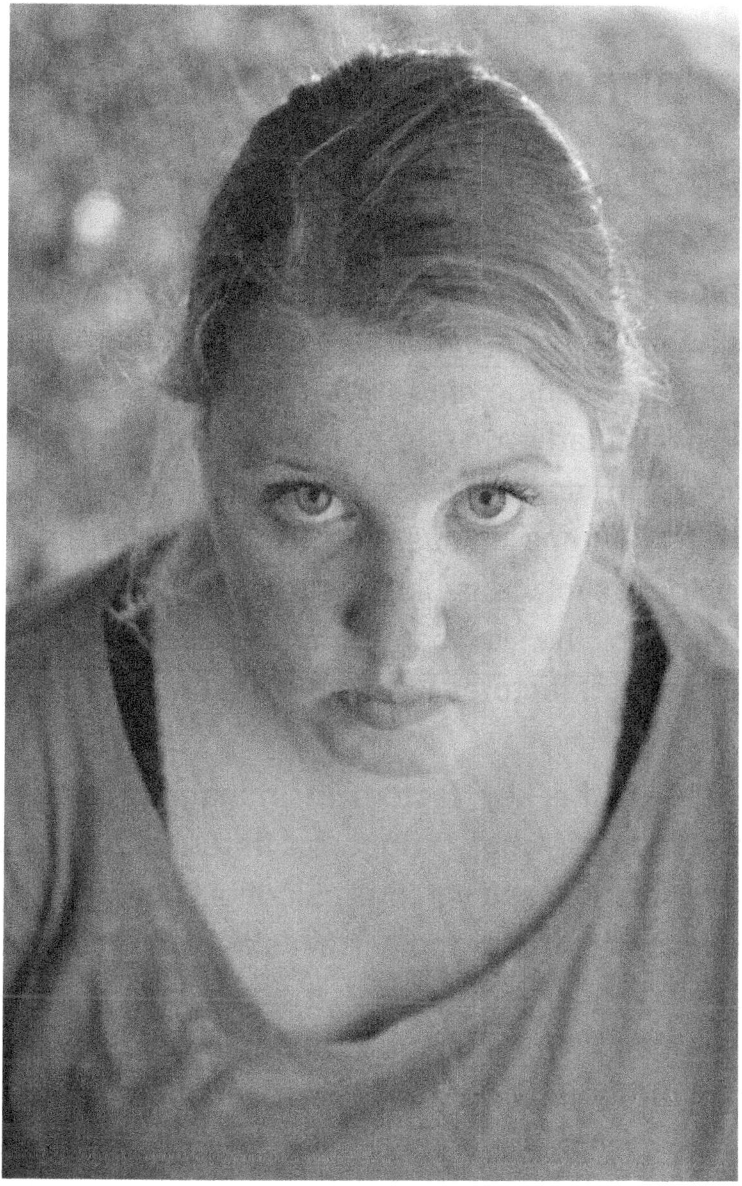

Chapter 1

Understanding Rosacea

What is Rosacea?

Rosacea is a chronic skin condition that affects millions of people around the world. It is characterized by redness, flushing, and visible blood vessels on the face, particularly on the cheeks, nose, chin, and forehead. In some cases, rosacea can also cause small, red bumps or pustules to appear on the skin. While the exact cause of rosacea is unknown, it is believed to be a combination of genetic and environmental factors.

One of the key factors in managing rosacea is understanding what triggers flare-ups. Common triggers include spicy foods, alcohol, hot beverages, sun exposure, stress, and certain skincare products. By identifying and avoiding these triggers, individuals with rosacea can help reduce the frequency and severity of their symptoms. Additionally, maintaining a healthy lifestyle, including regular exercise, adequate sleep, and a balanced diet, can also help improve overall skin health and reduce inflammation.

Many people with rosacea turn to natural remedies to help manage their symptoms. These can include dietary changes, such as eliminating trigger foods and incorporating anti-inflammatory foods like leafy greens, berries, and fatty fish. Herbal supplements, such as turmeric, licorice root, and green tea, are also commonly used to help reduce inflammation and promote skin healing.

Additionally, topical treatments like aloe vera gel, chamomile tea compresses, and raw honey masks can help soothe irritated skin and reduce redness.

In addition to natural remedies, there are also medical treatments available for rosacea. These can include prescription medications like antibiotics, topical creams, and laser therapy. It is important for individuals with rosacea to work closely with a dermatologist or healthcare provider to develop a treatment plan that is tailored to their specific needs and concerns. By combining natural remedies with medical treatments, individuals with rosacea can achieve clearer, healthier skin and improve their overall quality of life.

Overall, managing rosacea requires a holistic approach that addresses both the physical and emotional aspects of the condition. By understanding what rosacea is, identifying triggers, incorporating natural remedies, and seeking medical treatment when necessary, individuals with rosacea can take control of their skin health and achieve long-lasting results.

With dedication and patience, it is possible to heal rosacea naturally and enjoy clear, beautiful skin.

Common Triggers of Rosacea Flare-Ups

Rosacea is a chronic skin condition that can be triggered by a variety of factors, leading to flare-ups that can be both uncomfortable and embarrassing. In order to effectively manage your rosacea, it is important to identify and avoid these common triggers. By understanding what causes your flare-ups, you can take steps to minimize their impact on your skin and overall well-being.

One of the most common triggers of rosacea flare-ups is exposure to sunlight. UV rays can cause inflammation in the skin, leading to redness and irritation. It is important to protect your skin by wearing sunscreen with a high SPF, avoiding prolonged sun exposure, and wearing a wide-brimmed hat when outdoors. By taking these precautions, you can help prevent flare-ups caused by sun exposure.

Another common trigger of rosacea flare-ups is hot or spicy foods and beverages. These can cause blood vessels to dilate, leading to increased redness and flushing. If you notice that certain foods or drinks exacerbate your rosacea symptoms, try to avoid them or limit your intake. Opt for milder options and pay attention to how your skin reacts to different foods to help identify triggers.

Stress is another major trigger of rosacea flare-ups. When we are stressed, our bodies release hormones that can exacerbate inflammation in the skin. Finding healthy ways to manage stress, such as meditation, yoga, or deep breathing exercises, can help reduce the frequency and severity of flare-ups. It is also important to prioritize self-care and make time for activities that help you relax and unwind.

In addition to external triggers, internal factors such as hormonal changes can also contribute to rosacea flare-ups. Women may notice that their symptoms worsen during certain times of the month, or during pregnancy or menopause.

By tracking your symptoms and hormone levels, you may be able to identify patterns and take steps to manage your flare-ups. Consulting with a healthcare provider or dermatologist can also help you develop a treatment plan that addresses hormonal imbalances.

Overall, understanding and avoiding common triggers of rosacea flare-ups is key to managing this chronic skin condition. By taking a holistic approach to your skincare routine, diet, and lifestyle, you can help minimize flare-ups and achieve clearer, healthier skin.

Remember that everyone's triggers may be different, so it is important to pay attention to your own skin and how it responds to various factors. With patience and diligence, you can find a solution that works for you and helps you heal your rosacea naturally.

Types of Rosacea

In order to effectively manage rosacea, it is important to understand the different types of rosacea that can manifest on the skin. There are four main types of rosacea, each with its own unique set of symptoms and triggers. By identifying which type of rosacea you have, you can tailor your treatment plan to address your specific needs.

The 1st type rosacea is erythematotelangiectatic rosacea, which is characterized by persistent redness and visible blood vessels on the face. This type of rosacea can be triggered by factors such as sun exposure, hot drinks, spicy foods, and extreme temperatures. To manage erythematotelangiectatic rosacea, it is important to avoid these triggers, use gentle skincare products, and protect your skin from the sun.

The second type of rosacea is papulopustular rosacea, which presents as red bumps and pus-filled pimples on the skin. This type of rosacea is often mistaken for acne, but it is important to treat it differently in order to avoid exacerbating the condition.

To manage papulopustular rosacea, it is important to use gentle, non-comedogenic skincare products, avoid harsh ingredients, and consult with a dermatologist for personalized treatment options.

The third type of rosacea is phymatous rosacea, which is characterized by thickening skin and enlargement of the nose, chin, forehead, or ears. This type of rosacea is more common in men and can be difficult to treat without professional intervention. To manage phymatous rosacea, it is important to seek treatment from a dermatologist, who may recommend oral medications, laser therapy, or surgery to improve the appearance of the affected areas.

The fourth type of rosacea is ocular rosacea, which affects the eyes and eyelids and can cause symptoms such as redness, dryness, irritation, and sensitivity to light. Ocular rosacea can be uncomfortable and impact your quality of life, so it is important to seek treatment from an ophthalmologist or dermatologist who specializes in treating this condition. To manage ocular rosacea, it is important to use preservative-free eye drops, avoid rubbing your eyes, and protect your eyes from irritants such as smoke and wind.

By understanding the different types of rosacea and their unique symptoms and triggers, you can take proactive steps to manage your condition and improve the health and appearance of your skin. Remember to consult with a healthcare professional for personalized treatment options and guidance on how to heal rosacea naturally.

Symptoms of Rosacea

Rosacea is a chronic skin condition that affects millions of people worldwide. It is characterized by redness, flushing, and sometimes small, red bumps on the face. If you have rosacea, you may have noticed that your symptoms tend to come and go, often triggered by certain factors such as stress, spicy foods, alcohol, or extreme temperatures. Understanding the symptoms of rosacea is the first step in managing and treating this condition effectively.

One of the most common symptoms of rosacea is persistent facial redness, especially on the cheeks, nose, forehead, and chin. This redness may come and go, but for many people with rosacea, it is a constant presence.

In some cases, the redness may be accompanied by a feeling of warmth or burning in the affected areas. This can be frustrating and embarrassing, leading many individuals to seek out ways to cover up or reduce the redness.

Another symptom of rosacea is flushing, which is a sudden and temporary redness of the face that can be triggered by various factors such as stress, heat, or certain foods. Flushing episodes can be intense and may last for several minutes to hours. Some people with rosacea also experience small, red bumps or pimples on their face, which can be mistaken for acne. These bumps may be filled with pus and can be painful or itchy.

In more severe cases of rosacea, individuals may develop visible blood vessels on their face, known as telangiectasia. These blood vessels are often seen on the cheeks, nose, and chin and can give the skin a flushed or spider-like appearance. In rare cases, some people with rosacea may also experience eye symptoms, such as redness, dryness, itching, or a gritty sensation in the eyes. This condition, known as ocular rosacea, requires prompt treatment by an eye doctor.

If you are experiencing any of these symptoms, it is important to seek the advice of a dermatologist or skincare professional who can help you identify and manage your rosacea. While there is no cure for rosacea, there are many natural and holistic approaches that can help reduce redness, inflammation, and other symptoms associated with this condition. By taking a proactive approach to managing your rosacea, you can improve the health and appearance of your skin and feel more confident in your own skin.

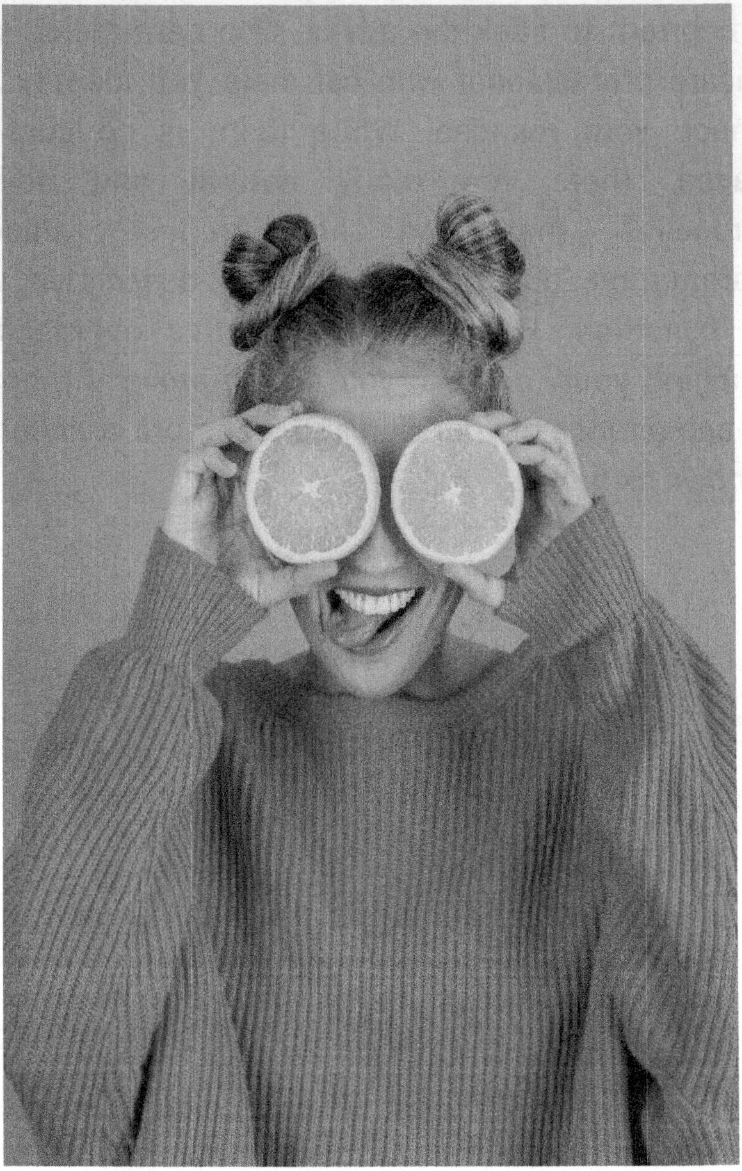

Chapter 2

The Holistic Approach to Healing Rosacea

Treating Rosacea from the Inside Out

Rosacea is a chronic skin condition that affects millions of people worldwide. While there is no cure for rosacea, there are ways to manage and treat the symptoms effectively. One approach that has gained popularity in recent years is treating rosacea from the inside out. This holistic approach focuses on addressing the root causes of rosacea, rather than just treating the symptoms on the surface.

One of the key components of treating rosacea from the inside out is paying attention to your diet. Certain foods and beverages can trigger flare-ups in individuals with rosacea, so it's important to identify and avoid these triggers. Common triggers include spicy foods, alcohol, caffeine, and dairy products. By eliminating these triggers from your diet, you may be able to reduce the frequency and severity of your flare-ups.

In addition to diet, stress management is also crucial in treating rosacea holistically. Stress is a common trigger for rosacea flare-ups, so finding ways to relax and unwind can greatly benefit your skin.

Techniques such as meditation, yoga, and deep breathing exercises can help to reduce stress levels and improve overall skin health. It's important to find what works best for you and incorporate stress management techniques into your daily routine.

Another important aspect of treating rosacea from the inside out is addressing any underlying health issues that may be contributing to your skin condition. Conditions such as gut dysbiosis, hormonal imbalances, and food sensitivities can all play a role in the development of rosacea.

By working with a healthcare provider to identify and address these underlying issues, you may be able to improve your skin health and reduce the severity of your symptoms.

In addition to diet, stress management, and addressing underlying health issues, incorporating natural remedies into your skincare routine can also help to manage rosacea symptoms. Ingredients such as green tea extract, aloe vera, and chamomile have anti-inflammatory properties that can help to soothe redness and irritation.

By taking a holistic approach to treating rosacea, you can improve your skin health from the inside out and achieve clear, radiant skin.

Importance of Diet and Nutrition

In the quest for clear and healthy skin, diet and nutrition play a crucial role, especially for those suffering from rosacea. The foods we eat can either exacerbate or alleviate the symptoms of this chronic skin condition. By understanding the importance of diet and nutrition, individuals with rosacea can take proactive steps towards healing their skin naturally.

One of the key reasons why diet and nutrition are essential for managing rosacea is that certain foods can trigger flare-ups and worsen symptoms. Common triggers include spicy foods, alcohol, caffeine, and high-acid foods like citrus fruits. By avoiding these triggers and opting for a diet rich in anti-inflammatory foods, individuals can reduce inflammation in the body and improve the overall health of their skin.

In addition to avoiding trigger foods, incorporating skin-friendly nutrients into your diet can help support the healing process. Foods rich in antioxidants, such as berries, leafy greens, and nuts, can help reduce oxidative stress and protect the skin from damage. Omega-3 fatty acids found in fatty fish, flaxseeds, and walnuts can also help reduce inflammation and improve skin health.

Furthermore, maintaining a balanced and varied diet can support gut health, which is closely linked to skin health. Probiotic-rich foods like yogurt, kefir, and sauerkraut can help promote a healthy gut microbiome, which in turn can improve the skin's barrier function and reduce inflammation.

By nourishing your body from the inside out, you can support your skin's natural healing process and reduce the frequency and severity of rosacea flare-ups.

In conclusion, the importance of diet and nutrition in managing rosacea cannot be overstated. By being mindful of trigger foods, incorporating skin-friendly nutrients, and supporting gut health, individuals with rosacea can take proactive steps towards healing their skin naturally. With a holistic approach to skincare that includes attention to diet and nutrition, individuals can achieve clear, healthy skin and reduce the impact of this chronic skin condition on their daily lives.

Stress Management Techniques

Living with rosacea can be challenging, especially when stress exacerbates symptoms. Stress is a common trigger for rosacea flare-ups, so it is important to incorporate stress management techniques into your daily routine. By learning how to effectively manage stress, you can improve your overall well-being and potentially reduce the frequency and severity of your rosacea symptoms.

One effective stress management technique is mindfulness meditation. By practicing mindfulness, you can learn to become more aware of your thoughts and emotions, and develop the ability to respond to stress in a calm and controlled manner. Mindfulness meditation can help you to stay present in the moment, rather than getting caught up in worries about the future or regrets about the past.

Another helpful stress management technique is deep breathing exercises. When you are feeling stressed, take a few moments to focus on your breath. Inhale deeply through your nose, hold for a few seconds, and then exhale slowly through your mouth. This simple practice can help to calm your nervous system and reduce feelings of anxiety and tension.

Engaging in regular physical activity is also a great way to manage stress and improve your overall health. Exercise releases endorphins, which are natural mood-boosting chemicals that can help to reduce stress and promote feelings of well-being. Whether you prefer yoga, walking, or dancing, finding a form of exercise that you enjoy can be a fun and effective way to manage stress.

Lastly, make sure to prioritize self-care and relaxation in your daily routine. Take time for yourself each day to engage in activities that bring you joy and relaxation, such as reading a book, taking a bath, or practicing a hobby. By taking care of your mental and emotional well-being, you can better manage stress and improve your skin health. By incorporating these stress management techniques into your daily routine, you can help to reduce the impact of stress on your rosacea symptoms and improve your overall quality of life.

Incorporating Exercise for Healthy Skin

Exercise is not only crucial for maintaining a healthy body, but it can also have a significant impact on the health of your skin, especially if you have rosacea. Regular physical activity helps to improve blood circulation, which can promote the delivery of essential nutrients and oxygen to the skin. This can lead to a healthier complexion and reduce the appearance of redness and inflammation associated with rosacea.

When incorporating exercise into your routine, it is important to choose activities that are gentle on the skin and unlikely to trigger flare-ups. Low-impact exercises such as walking, swimming, and yoga are excellent choices for individuals with rosacea. These activities can help to reduce stress levels, which is a common trigger for rosacea flare-ups, while also promoting overall skin health.

In addition to choosing the right types of exercise, it is also important to pay attention to your skincare routine before and after physical activity. Make sure to cleanse your skin before working out to remove any makeup or impurities that could clog pores and exacerbate rosacea symptoms.

After exercising, be sure to cleanse your skin again to remove sweat and bacteria that can contribute to flare-ups.

It is also important to stay hydrated before, during, and after exercise to keep your skin healthy and hydrated. Drinking plenty of water helps to flush out toxins from the body and can prevent dehydration, which can lead to dry, irritated skin.

Additionally, incorporating foods rich in antioxidants, such as fruits and vegetables, into your diet can help to protect your skin from damage caused by free radicals generated during exercise.

Overall, incorporating exercise into your routine can have numerous benefits for individuals with rosacea. By choosing gentle, low-impact activities, paying attention to your skincare routine, staying hydrated, and eating a healthy diet, you can promote healthier skin and reduce the frequency and severity of rosacea flare-ups. Remember to listen to your body and make adjustments to your exercise routine as needed to ensure that your skin remains healthy and radiant.

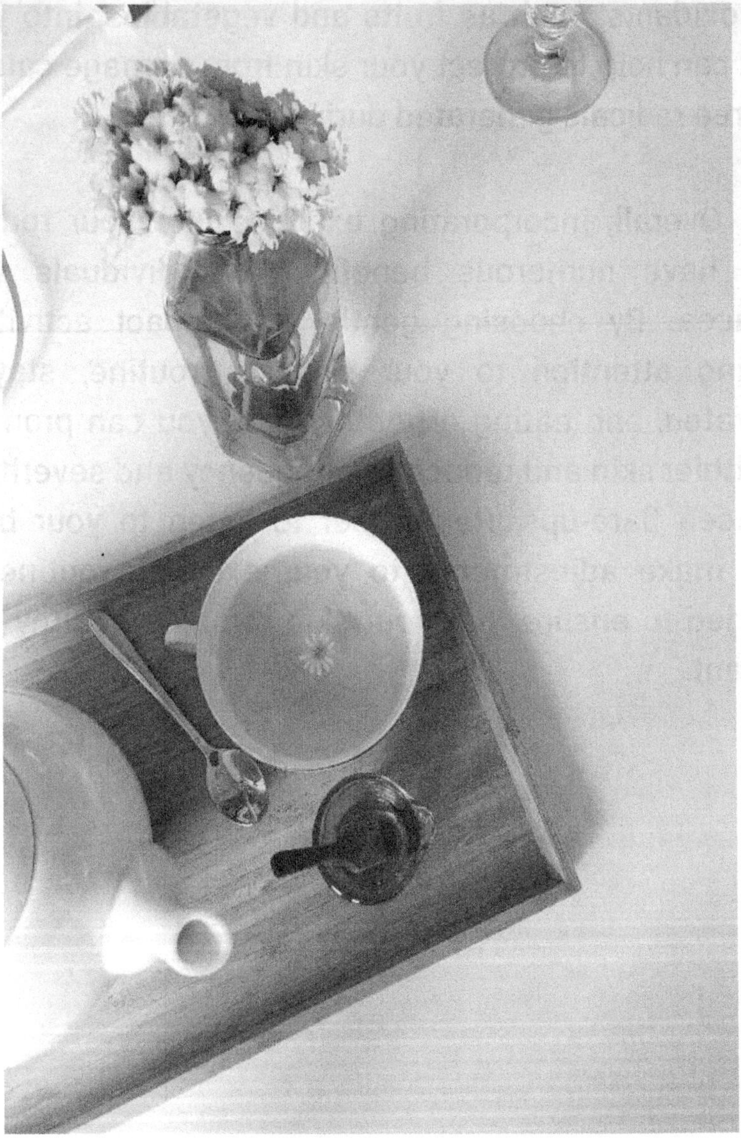

Chapter 3

Natural Remedies for Rosacea

Herbal Remedies for Rosacea

Herbal remedies have long been used to treat various skin conditions, including rosacea. Many people who suffer from rosacea have found relief from their symptoms by incorporating herbal remedies into their skincare routine. In this subchapter, we will explore some of the most effective herbal remedies for rosacea and how they can help improve the appearance of your skin.

One of the most popular herbal remedies for rosacea is green tea. Green tea is rich in antioxidants and anti-inflammatory properties, which can help reduce redness and inflammation associated with rosacea. You can apply green tea topically to your skin or drink it as a tea to reap its benefits. Many people have found that incorporating green tea into their daily routine has helped improve the overall health and appearance of their skin.

Another effective herbal remedy for rosacea is licorice root. Licorice root contains compounds that have anti-inflammatory and skin-soothing properties, making it a great option for calming redness and irritation associated with rosacea. You can find licorice root in skincare products or create your own DIY mask using licorice root powder mixed with water. Many people have reported significant improvements in their rosacea symptoms after using licorice root regularly.

Chamomile is another herbal remedy that can help soothe and calm inflamed skin caused by rosacea. Chamomile has anti-inflammatory and anti-bacterial properties, making it an excellent option for reducing redness and irritation.

You can use chamomile tea bags as a compress on your skin or incorporate chamomile extract into your skincare routine. Many people have found that chamomile not only helps improve the appearance of their skin but also reduces the frequency and severity of rosacea flare-ups.

In addition to green tea, licorice root, and chamomile, other herbal remedies that may help improve rosacea symptoms include aloe vera, calendula, and lavender. These herbs have soothing and anti-inflammatory properties that can help reduce redness, inflammation, and irritation associated with rosacea.

You can find skincare products containing these herbal ingredients or create your own DIY treatments at home. Incorporating herbal remedies into your skincare routine can help improve the overall health and appearance of your skin, providing relief from the symptoms of rosacea.

Overall, herbal remedies can be a natural and effective way to manage rosacea symptoms and improve the appearance of your skin. By incorporating herbs like green tea, licorice root, chamomile, aloe vera, calendula, and lavender into your skincare routine, you may find relief from redness, inflammation, and irritation associated with rosacea. Remember to consult with a healthcare professional or skincare specialist before trying any new herbal remedies to ensure they are safe and suitable for your skin type.

Essential Oils for Rosacea

Rosacea is a common skin condition that affects millions of people worldwide. Characterized by redness, flushing, and sometimes pustules on the face, rosacea can be both physically and emotionally challenging to deal with. While there are various treatment options available, many people are turning to natural remedies, such as essential oils, to help manage their symptoms.

Essential oils are highly concentrated plant extracts that have been used for centuries for their therapeutic properties. When it comes to rosacea, certain essential oils have been found to be particularly beneficial in soothing inflammation, reducing redness, and promoting overall skin health. Some of the most effective essential oils for rosacea include lavender, chamomile, tea tree, and helichrysum.

Lavender essential oil is known for its calming and anti-inflammatory properties, making it an excellent choice for those with rosacea. Chamomile essential oil is also highly soothing and can help reduce redness and irritation.

Tea tree essential oil has powerful antibacterial and anti-inflammatory properties, making it effective in treating the pustules that can sometimes accompany rosacea. Helichrysum essential oil is another great option for rosacea, as it can help promote healing and reduce inflammation.

When using essential oils for rosacea, it is important to dilute them properly before applying them to the skin. This can be done by mixing a few drops of the essential oil with a carrier oil, such as jojoba or coconut oil. It is also recommended to do a patch test before using any new essential oil to ensure that you do not have an allergic reaction.

In conclusion, essential oils can be a valuable addition to your holistic approach to managing rosacea. By incorporating these natural remedies into your skincare routine, you may find relief from your symptoms and enjoy clearer, healthier skin. Remember to always consult with a healthcare professional before trying any new treatment, and listen to your body to determine what works best for you.

Homeopathic Treatments for Rosacea

Rosacea is a common skin condition that affects millions of people worldwide. Characterized by redness, flushing, and pimple-like bumps on the face, rosacea can be both physically and emotionally distressing. While there is no known cure for rosacea, there are several homeopathic treatments that can help manage symptoms and improve the overall health of your skin.

One of the most popular homeopathic treatments for rosacea is sulfur. Sulfur is a naturally occurring mineral that has been used for centuries to treat various skin conditions, including rosacea. When applied topically, sulfur can help reduce inflammation, redness, and irritation associated with rosacea. It also has antibacterial properties that can help prevent infection and promote healing of the skin.

Another effective homeopathic treatment for rosacea is chamomile. Chamomile is known for its calming and anti-inflammatory properties, making it an ideal treatment for sensitive and inflamed skin.

You can use chamomile tea as a toner or apply chamomile essential oil diluted in a carrier oil directly to the affected areas. Chamomile can help reduce redness, soothe irritation, and promote healing of the skin.

Calendula is another homeopathic remedy that can help relieve symptoms of rosacea. Calendula is a plant that has been used for centuries to treat various skin conditions, including rosacea. It has anti-inflammatory and antiseptic properties that can help reduce redness, swelling, and irritation associated with rosacea. You can find calendula creams, ointments, and tinctures at most health food stores or online.

In addition to topical treatments, there are several dietary changes you can make to help manage rosacea naturally. Avoiding trigger foods such as spicy foods, alcohol, and caffeine can help reduce flare-ups and improve the overall health of your skin. Incorporating anti-inflammatory foods such as leafy greens, fatty fish, and berries into your diet can also help reduce inflammation and promote healing of the skin.

Overall, homeopathic treatments can be a safe and effective way to manage rosacea naturally. By incorporating sulfur, chamomile, calendula, and making dietary changes into your skincare routine, you can help reduce redness, inflammation, and irritation associated with rosacea. Remember to consult with a healthcare professional before starting any new treatment regimen, especially if you are pregnant, nursing, or have underlying health conditions.

DIY Skincare Recipes for Rosacea

Are you tired of trying expensive skincare products that promise to alleviate your rosacea symptoms, only to be left disappointed with minimal results? Look no further - in this subchapter, we will explore DIY skincare recipes specifically tailored for individuals with rosacea.

By using natural ingredients that are gentle on sensitive skin, you can soothe inflammation, reduce redness, and promote overall skin health without breaking the bank.

One of the most effective DIY skincare recipes for rosacea is a soothing oatmeal mask. Oatmeal is known for its anti-inflammatory properties, making it perfect for calming redness and irritation associated with rosacea.

Simply mix ground oats with water to form a paste, apply to clean skin, and leave on for 15-20 minutes before rinsing off. This mask can be used weekly to help improve the appearance of rosacea-prone skin.

Another great DIY recipe for rosacea is a homemade toner using apple cider vinegar. Apple cider vinegar has antibacterial and anti-inflammatory properties that can help to balance the skin's pH levels and reduce redness.

Mix equal parts apple cider vinegar and water, apply to a cotton pad, and gently swipe over the face after cleansing. This toner can be used daily to help soothe and tone rosacea-affected skin.

For those with rosacea, it is essential to nourish the skin with hydrating ingredients that won't trigger flare-ups. A DIY moisturizer using aloe vera gel and coconut oil is a great option for soothing and moisturizing sensitive skin.

Mix equal parts aloe vera gel and coconut oil, apply to the skin, and gently massage in until fully absorbed. This moisturizer can be used daily to keep the skin hydrated and calm.

In addition to topical treatments, it is important to support the skin from the inside out. A DIY green smoothie containing ingredients like kale, spinach, cucumber, and avocado can provide the skin with essential vitamins and nutrients to promote healing and reduce inflammation.

By incorporating this nutrient-rich smoothie into your daily routine, you can help to improve the overall health of your skin and minimize rosacea symptoms.

In conclusion, taking a holistic approach to skincare by incorporating DIY recipes tailored for rosacea can help to improve the appearance and health of your skin naturally. By using gentle, natural ingredients that are suited for sensitive skin, you can soothe inflammation, reduce redness, and promote overall skin health without harsh chemicals or irritants. Try incorporating these DIY skincare recipes into your routine and see the difference they can make in managing your rosacea symptoms.

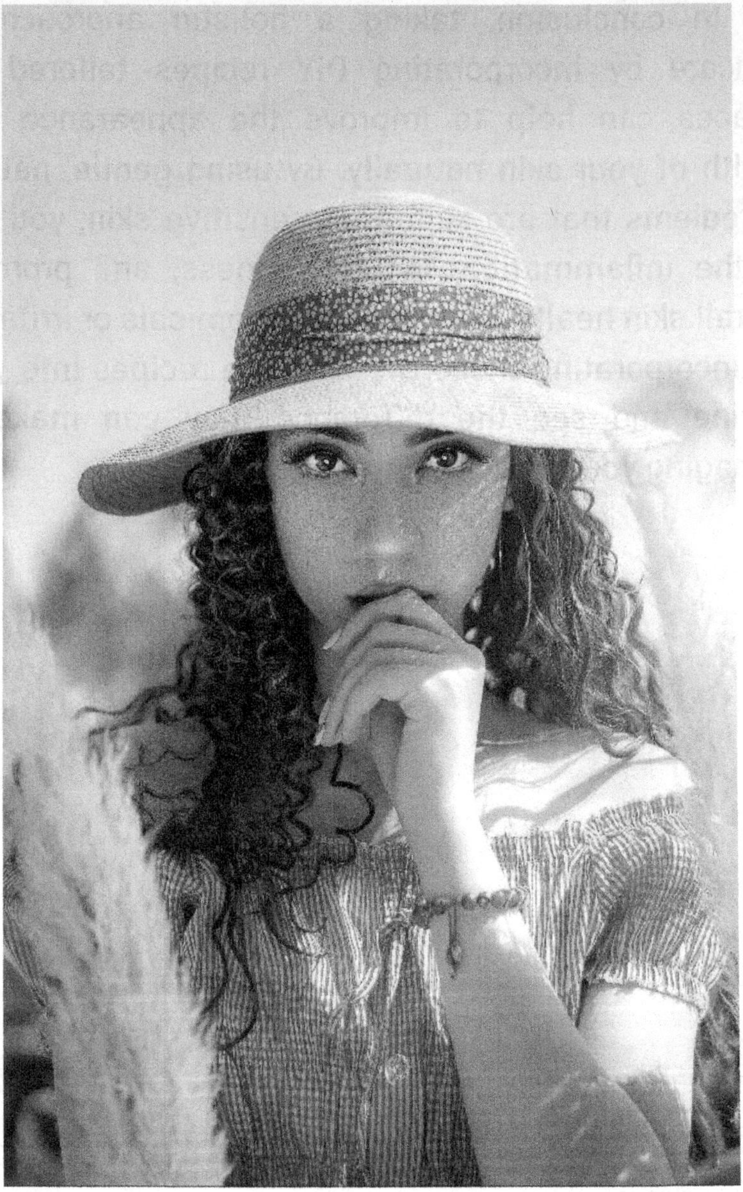

Chapter 4

Lifestyle Changes for Managing Rosacea

Skincare Routine for Rosacea

If you suffer from rosacea, you know how frustrating and embarrassing it can be to deal with flare-ups and redness on a daily basis. However, with the right skincare routine, you can manage your symptoms and improve the overall health of your skin. In this subchapter, we will discuss the best practices for creating a skincare routine specifically tailored to individuals with rosacea.

The first step in any skincare routine for rosacea is to use gentle, non-irritating products. Look for cleansers, moisturizers, and other skincare products that are free of harsh chemicals and fragrances. These can trigger flare-ups and worsen your symptoms. Opt for products that are specifically formulated for sensitive skin and contain soothing ingredients like aloe vera, chamomile, and oatmeal.

It is also important to cleanse your skin gently and thoroughly. Use a mild, non-abrasive cleanser to remove dirt, oil, and makeup without stripping your skin of its natural oils. Avoid scrubbing or rubbing your skin too harshly, as this can aggravate rosacea symptoms. Instead, use gentle, circular motions to cleanse your skin and pat it dry with a soft towel.

In addition to cleansing, moisturizing is crucial for maintaining healthy skin when you have rosacea. Look for a lightweight, non-comedogenic moisturizer that will hydrate your skin without clogging your pores. Moisturizing regularly will help to soothe and protect your skin, reducing redness and irritation. Be sure to apply moisturizer both in the morning and at night to keep your skin hydrated and balanced.

Finally, it is important to protect your skin from the sun, as UV rays can trigger rosacea flare-ups. Use a broad-spectrum sunscreen with an SPF of 30 or higher every day, even on cloudy days. Additionally, wear a wide-brimmed hat and sunglasses to shield your face from the sun's harmful rays.

By following these simple steps and creating a skincare routine tailored to your specific needs, you can effectively manage your rosacea symptoms and achieve clear, healthy skin.

Sun Protection and Rosacea

Sun protection is crucial for individuals with rosacea, as exposure to the sun's harmful UV rays can exacerbate symptoms and trigger flare-ups. It is important for those with rosacea to use a broad-spectrum sunscreen with an SPF of 30 or higher every day, even on cloudy days.

Additionally, wearing protective clothing such as hats and sunglasses can help shield the skin from the sun's damaging effects. By incorporating sun protection into their daily routine, individuals with rosacea can help prevent further irritation and maintain healthier skin.

In addition to sunscreen, seeking shade and avoiding direct sunlight during peak hours can also help protect the skin from sun damage. This is especially important for individuals with rosacea, as their skin is more sensitive and prone to reactions.

By being mindful of sun exposure and taking steps to limit it, those with rosacea can help prevent flare-ups and maintain smoother, clearer skin.

It is important for individuals with rosacea to choose sunscreens that are non-comedogenic and fragrance-free to avoid further irritation. Look for sunscreens that contain zinc oxide or titanium dioxide, as these ingredients are less likely to cause stinging or burning on sensitive skin. Additionally, opting for mineral sunscreens over chemical sunscreens can help reduce the risk of irritation and flare-ups in individuals with rosacea.

Incorporating sun protection into a holistic approach to managing rosacea is essential for maintaining healthy skin and minimizing symptoms. By combining sun protection with other natural remedies and lifestyle changes, individuals with rosacea can work towards healing their skin from the inside out. By taking a proactive approach to sun protection and overall skin health, individuals with rosacea can experience improved skin clarity and reduced flare-ups over time.

In conclusion, sun protection plays a crucial role in managing rosacea and preventing flare-ups. By incorporating daily sunscreen use, seeking shade, and choosing skin-friendly sunscreens, individuals with rosacea can help protect their skin from the sun's harmful rays and maintain healthier skin. By taking a holistic approach to managing rosacea that includes sun protection, individuals can work towards clearer, smoother skin and improved overall skin health.

Makeup Tips for Rosacea

If you have rosacea, you may feel self-conscious about the redness and bumps that can appear on your skin. However, with the right makeup tips, you can help minimize the appearance of your rosacea and feel more confident in your skin. In this subchapter, we will discuss some helpful makeup tips for rosacea that can help you achieve a flawless look.

First and foremost, it is important to start with a clean and moisturized face. Make sure to use a gentle cleanser and a hydrating moisturizer that is suitable for sensitive skin. This will help create a smooth base for your makeup and prevent any irritation that could worsen your rosacea.

When choosing makeup products for rosacea, opt for ones that are fragrance-free, non-comedogenic, and specifically formulated for sensitive skin. Look for products that contain soothing ingredients like aloe vera, chamomile, and green tea, which can help calm redness and inflammation. Avoid products that contain alcohol, which can be drying and irritating to the skin.

When applying foundation, use a light hand and opt for a formula that provides buildable coverage. Avoid heavy, full-coverage foundations that can exacerbate the appearance of rosacea. Instead, choose a lightweight, mineral-based foundation that allows your skin to breathe and provides a natural finish. Use a damp makeup sponge or brush to blend the foundation seamlessly into your skin.

To conceal redness and bumps, use a color-correcting concealer in a green or yellow shade. These colors can help neutralize the redness in your skin and create a more even complexion. Apply the concealer sparingly to the areas where you need it most, such as around your nose and cheeks, and blend it out gently with your fingertips or a makeup brush.

Finish off your makeup look with a setting spray to help lock everything in place and prevent your makeup from sliding off throughout the day. Look for a setting spray that is alcohol-free and formulated for sensitive skin. With these makeup tips for rosacea, you can enhance your natural beauty and feel more confident in your skin.

Seeking Support and Resources for Rosacea

Seeking support and resources for rosacea can be a crucial step in managing this chronic skin condition. While there is no cure for rosacea, there are many ways to alleviate symptoms and improve the overall health of your skin. By seeking out support from others who have rosacea, you can gain valuable insights and tips for managing your condition effectively.

One of the best resources for people with rosacea is the National Rosacea Society (NRS). This organization provides valuable information on rosacea, including tips for managing symptoms, treatment options, and support groups.

By joining the NRS, you can connect with others who have rosacea and learn from their experiences.

In addition to seeking support from organizations like the NRS, it is also important to seek out resources for natural healing methods for rosacea. Many people with rosacea find relief from their symptoms by using natural remedies such as aloe vera, green tea, and honey. These natural ingredients have anti-inflammatory and soothing properties that can help to calm irritated skin and reduce redness.

Another valuable resource for people with rosacea is a holistic skincare practitioner. These professionals can provide personalized recommendations for managing rosacea symptoms based on your individual needs and lifestyle. By working with a holistic skincare practitioner, you can develop a customized treatment plan that addresses the root causes of your rosacea and promotes overall skin health.

In conclusion, seeking support and resources for rosacea is an important step in managing this chronic skin condition. By connecting with others who have rosacea, exploring natural healing methods, and working with a holistic skincare practitioner, you can take control of your rosacea and improve the health of your skin. Remember that everyone's experience with rosacea is unique, so it may take some trial and error to find the best approach for managing your symptoms. Stay positive, stay informed, and don't be afraid to seek out the support you need to achieve clear, healthy skin.

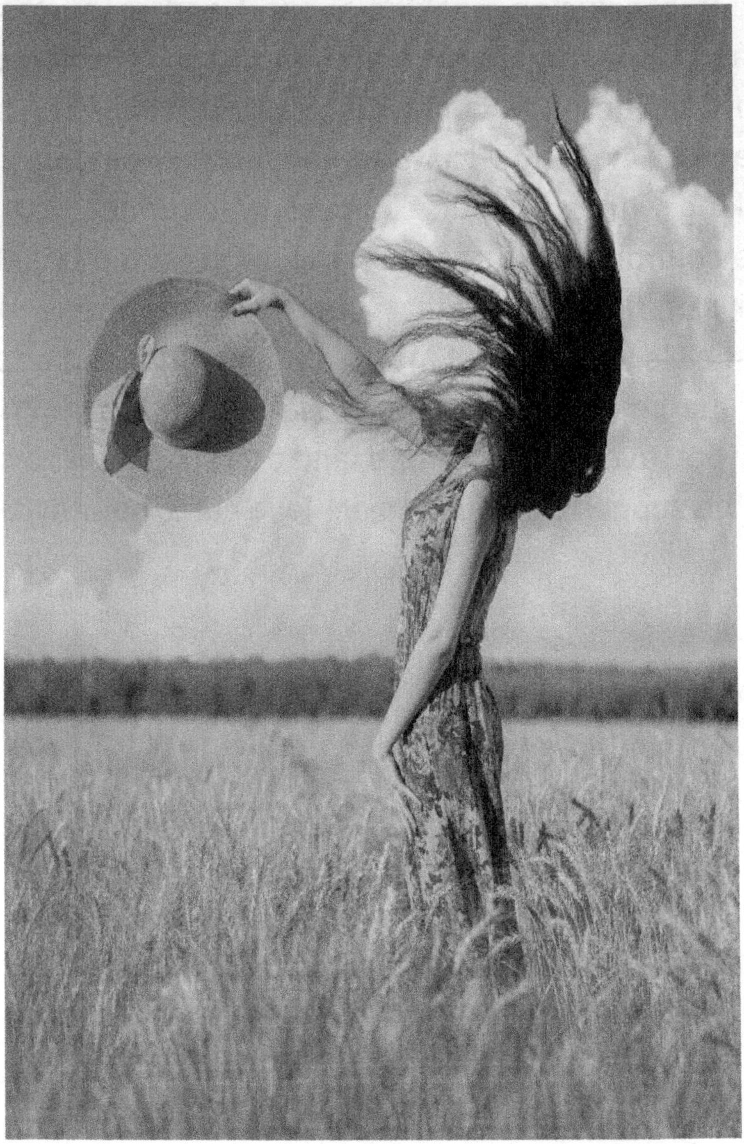

Chapter 5

Maintaining Clear Skin and Preventing Flare-Ups

Monitoring Triggers and Symptoms

One of the most important aspects of managing rosacea is being able to identify and monitor your triggers and symptoms. By understanding what causes your flare-ups and recognizing the signs that your rosacea is worsening, you can take proactive steps to prevent and alleviate symptoms. It is crucial to keep a detailed journal of your daily activities, diet, skincare routine, and environmental factors to pinpoint potential triggers.

Common triggers for rosacea include spicy foods, hot beverages, alcohol, stress, extreme temperatures, and certain skincare products. By tracking your daily habits and noting any changes in your skin, you can start to identify patterns and make necessary adjustments to your lifestyle. This will not only help you prevent flare-ups but also improve the overall health of your skin.

Monitoring your symptoms is also key to managing rosacea effectively. Pay attention to any redness, flushing, bumps, or swelling on your face, as well as any discomfort or itching. By keeping a close eye on these symptoms, you can address them promptly and prevent them from escalating. It is important to consult with a healthcare professional if you notice any significant changes in your skin or if your symptoms become severe.

In addition to tracking your triggers and symptoms, it is essential to adopt a holistic approach to healing rosacea naturally. This includes making dietary changes, practicing stress-reducing techniques, using gentle skincare products, and protecting your skin from harsh environmental factors. By taking a comprehensive approach to managing your rosacea, you can improve the health and appearance of your skin from the inside out.

Overall, monitoring your triggers and symptoms is a crucial step in managing rosacea naturally. By being proactive and attentive to your skin's needs, you can minimize flare-ups, reduce symptoms, and achieve clear and healthy skin.

Remember to be patient and consistent in your approach, as healing rosacea naturally may take time but will ultimately lead to long-lasting results.

Regularly Assessing Skin Health

Regularly assessing your skin health is crucial when dealing with rosacea. By monitoring the condition of your skin on a regular basis, you can track any changes or flare-ups and take appropriate action to manage your symptoms effectively. One of the key aspects of assessing your skin health is to pay attention to any triggers that may exacerbate your rosacea. This can include factors such as certain foods, weather conditions, stress, or skincare products. By identifying and avoiding these triggers, you can help prevent flare-ups and maintain clearer skin.

It is also important to regularly assess the effectiveness of your current skincare routine and make adjustments as needed. This may involve consulting with a dermatologist or skincare specialist to determine the best products and treatments for your skin type and condition.

By keeping track of how your skin responds to different products and treatments, you can tailor your skincare regimen to suit your individual needs and achieve optimal results.

In addition to monitoring your skin health, it is essential to practice good skincare habits on a daily basis to help manage your rosacea. This includes cleansing your skin gently, using non-comedogenic products, and moisturizing regularly to maintain a healthy skin barrier. Regularly assessing the condition of your skin can help you identify any areas that may need extra attention and ensure that you are taking the necessary steps to keep your skin healthy and clear.

Another important aspect of assessing skin health is to pay attention to any changes in your skin's appearance or texture. This may include redness, bumps, dryness, or irritation, which can indicate a flare-up or reaction to a particular trigger. By monitoring these changes and seeking guidance from a healthcare professional, you can address any issues promptly and prevent them from worsening. Regularly assessing your skin health can help you stay proactive in managing your rosacea and achieving clearer, healthier skin.

Overall, regularly assessing your skin health is essential for managing rosacea and maintaining clear skin. By monitoring your skin for changes, identifying triggers, and adjusting your skincare routine as needed, you can take control of your condition and improve the overall health and appearance of your skin. By staying vigilant and proactive in caring for your skin, you can effectively manage your rosacea and achieve long-lasting results.

Building a Long-Term Plan for Rosacea Management

Building a long-term plan for rosacea management is crucial for those who suffer from this chronic skin condition. While there is no cure for rosacea, there are steps you can take to effectively manage your symptoms and improve the overall health of your skin. By implementing a holistic approach to clear skin, you can work towards healing your rosacea naturally and achieving long-lasting results.

One of the first steps in building a long-term plan for rosacea management is to identify and avoid triggers that exacerbate your symptoms. Common triggers include sun exposure, spicy foods, alcohol, stress, and certain skincare products. By keeping a journal and tracking your flare-ups, you can pinpoint which triggers affect your skin the most and make necessary adjustments to your daily routine.

In addition to avoiding triggers, it is important to establish a consistent skincare routine that caters to the specific needs of your rosacea-prone skin. This may include using gentle, non-irritating cleansers, moisturizers, and sunscreen that are free of harsh chemicals and fragrances. Incorporating natural remedies such as aloe vera, green tea, and chamomile can also help soothe and calm inflamed skin.

Furthermore, adopting a healthy lifestyle that includes regular exercise, a balanced diet, and stress management techniques can significantly improve the overall health of your skin. Exercise increases blood flow, which promotes healing and reduces inflammation, while a diet rich in antioxidants and omega-3 fatty acids can help nourish and protect your skin from within.

Stress management techniques such as yoga, meditation, and deep breathing exercises can also help reduce stress-related flare-ups.

By implementing these strategies and taking a holistic approach to clear skin, you can build a long-term plan for rosacea management that addresses the root causes of your symptoms and promotes healing from the inside out. With patience, consistency, and a commitment to self-care, you can achieve lasting results and enjoy healthier, clearer skin for years to come.

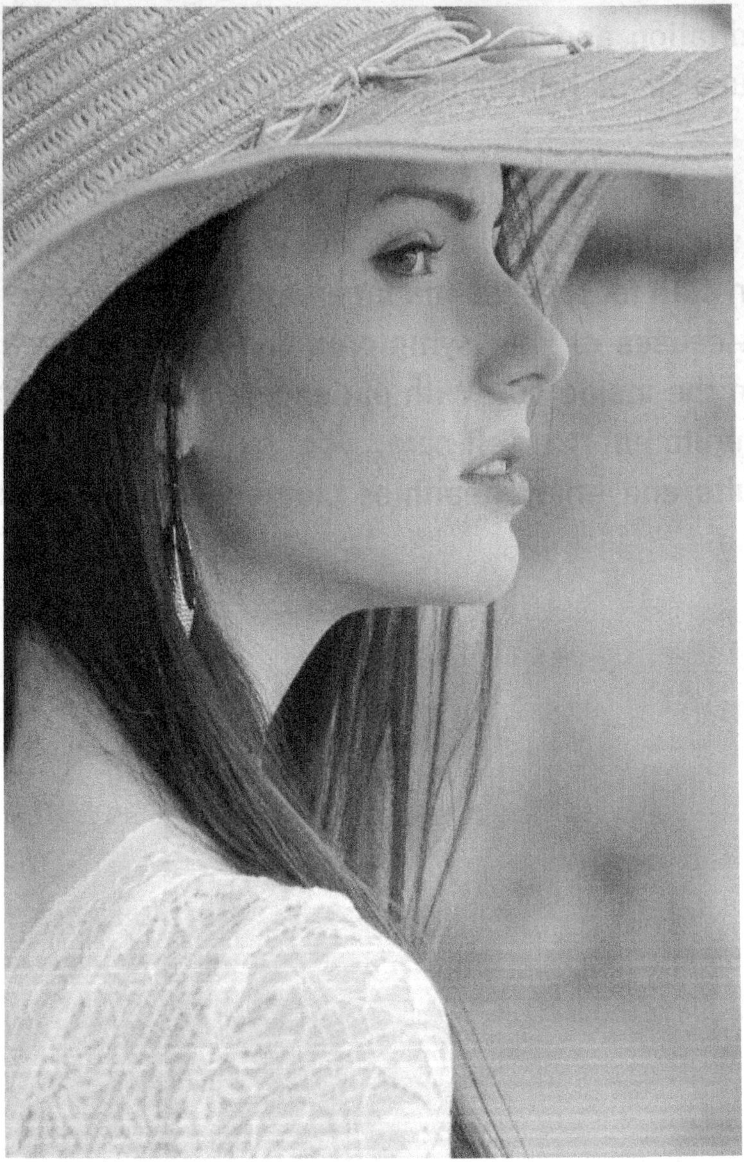

Chapter 6

Conclusion

Recap of Holistic Approaches to Clear Skin

In this subchapter, we will take a closer look at the holistic approaches to achieving clear, radiant skin for those suffering from rosacea. Rosacea is a chronic skin condition that causes redness, flushing, and sometimes acne-like bumps on the face. While there is no cure for rosacea, there are natural and holistic methods that can help manage symptoms and improve the overall health of your skin.

One of the key components of a holistic approach to clear skin is focusing on your diet. Certain foods can trigger flare-ups and worsen symptoms of rosacea. It is important to avoid spicy foods, alcohol, caffeine, and processed foods that can aggravate inflammation in the skin. Instead, opt for a diet rich in fruits, vegetables, whole grains, and lean proteins to support healthy skin function.

In addition to a healthy diet, stress management techniques are essential for those with rosacea. Stress can trigger flare-ups and exacerbate symptoms of rosacea. Practicing relaxation techniques such as deep breathing, meditation, and yoga can help calm the mind and body, reducing inflammation in the skin. Finding ways to reduce stress in your daily life can have a significant impact on the health of your skin.

Another important aspect of a holistic approach to clear skin is using natural skincare products. Many conventional skincare products contain harsh chemicals and irritants that can worsen symptoms of rosacea. Opt for gentle, natural products that are free of fragrances, dyes, and other potential triggers. Look for products that contain soothing ingredients such as aloe vera, chamomile, and green tea to help calm redness and inflammation.

In conclusion, taking a holistic approach to clear skin involves addressing the root causes of rosacea and supporting the overall health of your skin. By focusing on your diet, managing stress, and using natural skincare products, you can improve the appearance of your skin and reduce symptoms of rosacea.

Remember that everyone's skin is unique, so it may take some trial and error to find the best approach for your individual needs. With patience and persistence, you can achieve clear, radiant skin and manage your rosacea naturally.

Empowering Yourself to Take Control of Your Rosacea

Rosacea can be a frustrating and sometimes embarrassing condition to deal with, but it doesn't have to control your life. By empowering yourself to take control of your rosacea, you can make positive changes that will improve your skin and your overall well-being. Here are some tips to help you on your journey to clear skin.

First and foremost, it's important to educate yourself about rosacea. Understanding the triggers and symptoms of your condition can help you make informed decisions about your skincare routine and lifestyle choices. By learning more about rosacea, you can also feel more confident in discussing your condition with healthcare professionals and seeking the best treatment options for your specific needs.

One of the most empowering things you can do to take control of your rosacea is to adopt a holistic approach to skincare. This means focusing on not only treating the symptoms of your condition, but also addressing the underlying causes.

By incorporating natural remedies, such as a healthy diet, stress management techniques, and gentle skincare products, you can support your body's natural healing processes and promote clear, radiant skin from the inside out.

In addition to holistic skincare practices, it's important to prioritize self-care and stress management in your daily routine. Stress is a common trigger for rosacea flare-ups, so finding ways to relax and unwind can help prevent breakouts and improve the overall health of your skin.

Whether it's through meditation, yoga, exercise, or simply taking time for yourself each day, finding ways to reduce stress and prioritize self-care can have a significant impact on your rosacea symptoms.

Finally, remember that you are not alone in your struggle with rosacea. Connecting with others who have similar experiences can provide support, encouragement, and valuable insights into managing your condition. Whether it's through online forums, support groups, or speaking with a dermatologist who specializes in rosacea, reaching out to others for guidance and support can help you feel empowered and motivated on your journey to clear skin.

By taking control of your rosacea and adopting a holistic approach to skincare, you can make positive changes that will improve your skin and your overall well-being.

Moving Forward with Confidence and Knowledge

Moving forward with confidence and knowledge is essential for anyone dealing with rosacea. It can be a challenging condition to manage, but with the right tools and information, you can take control of your skin health and improve your overall well-being. By adopting a holistic approach to treating rosacea, you can address the root causes of the condition and work towards clear, healthy skin.

One of the first steps in moving forward with confidence and knowledge is understanding the triggers of your rosacea. By keeping a journal and tracking your symptoms, you can identify patterns and determine what may be exacerbating your condition. Common triggers include stress, certain foods, alcohol, and extreme temperatures. By pinpointing your triggers, you can make lifestyle adjustments to help manage your symptoms and prevent flare-ups.

Another important aspect of moving forward with confidence and knowledge is educating yourself about natural treatment options for rosacea. Many people find relief from their symptoms by using gentle, natural remedies such as aloe vera, green tea, and chamomile. These ingredients have anti-inflammatory properties that can help soothe redness and irritation, making them valuable additions to your skincare routine.

In addition to natural remedies, it's important to prioritize self-care and stress management when dealing with rosacea. Stress is a common trigger for flare-ups, so finding ways to relax and unwind can make a significant difference in your skin health.

Whether it's practicing yoga, meditating, or simply taking time for yourself, finding ways to reduce stress can help improve your overall well-being and reduce the severity of your symptoms.

By committing to a holistic approach to treating rosacea, you can move forward with confidence and knowledge, knowing that you are taking proactive steps to improve your skin health. By understanding your triggers, exploring natural treatment options, and prioritizing self-care, you can empower yourself to manage your condition effectively and achieve clear, healthy skin.

Remember, you are not alone in your journey – there are resources and support available to help you on your path to healing.

Author Notes & Acknowledgments

First and foremost, I would like to express my deepest gratitude to the people who inspired and supported me throughout the journey of writing this book. This project would not have been possible without their unwavering belief in me and their invaluable contributions.

To my wife, thank you for your constant encouragement and understanding. Your love and support have been my anchor during the challenging times of researching and writing this book. Your belief in my ability to make a difference in people's lives has been my driving force.

I would also like to disclose that this book contains some renewed artificial intelligence-generated content. I really appreciate very recent technological innovation by outstanding scientists and of course our reader's understanding.

Lastly, I want to express my deepest gratitude to the readers of this book. I sincerely hope the strategies and methods outlined within these pages will provide you with the knowledge and tools needed to truly make your life much better. Your commitment to seeking any good solutions and willingness to explore multiple methods is commendable.

Author Bio

Johnson Wu earned his MD in 1982. With over 40 years of clinical experience, he has worked in hospitals in Zhejiang and Shanghai, China, as well as the Royal Marsden Hospital (part of Imperial College) in London, UK.

Upon the recommendation of Sir Aaron Klug, the president of The Royal Society and a Nobel Prize winner in Chemistry, Dr. Wu was honorably awarded a British Royal Society Fellowship. He has published medical books and articles in seven countries and currently practices medicine in Canada.

Made in the USA
Monee, IL
04 November 2026

67379624R00039